The Sheldon Short Guide to
Depression

Dr Tim Cantopher studied at University College, London, and University College Hospital. He trained as a psychiatrist at St James' Hospital, Portsmouth, and St George's Hospital Medical School. He has been a member of the Royal College of Psychiatrists since 1983 and was elected fellow of the college in 1999. Before his retirement, Dr Cantopher worked as a consultant psychiatrist with the Priory Group of Hospitals for many years, and he has published a number of research projects across the field of psychiatry. He is the author of *Stress-related Illness* (2007) and *Dying for a Drink* (2011), both published by Sheldon Press. Dr Cantopher is married with three children.

D1650463

9 40247666

Sheldon Short Guides

A full list of titles in the Overcoming Common Problems
series is also available from Sheldon Press, 36 Causton Street,
London SW1P 4ST and on our website at
www.sheldonpress.co.uk

Depression
Dr Tim Cantopher

Memory Problems
Dr Sallie Baxendale

Phobias and Panic
Professor Kevin Gournay

Worry and Anxiety
Dr Frank Tallis

THE SHELDON SHORT GUIDE TO
DEPRESSION

Dr **Tim Cantopher**

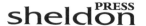

First published in Great Britain in 2015

Sheldon Press
36 Causton Street
London SW1P 4ST
www.sheldonpress.co.uk

British Library Cataloguing-in-Publication Data
A catalogue record for this book is available from the
British Library

ISBN 978-1-84709-370-7
eBook ISBN 978-1-84709-371-4

Typeset by Fakenham Prepress Solutions, Fakenham,
Norfolk NR21 8NN
First printed in Great Britain by Ashford Colour Press
Subsequently digitally reprinted in Great Britain

eBook by Fakenham Prepress Solutions, Fakenham,
Norfolk NR21 8NN

Produced on paper from sustainable forests

Contents

1

What is depressive illness?

Depressive illness is not a psychological or emotional state and is not a mental illness. It is not a form of madness. *It is a physical illness.*

This is not a metaphor; it is a fact. Clinical (severe, persistent) depression is every bit as physical a condition as pneumonia or a broken leg. If I were to perform a lumbar puncture on my patients (which, new patients of mine will be pleased to hear, I don't), I would be able to demonstrate in the chemical analysis of the cerebro-spinal fluid (the fluid around the brain and spine) a deficiency of two chemicals: serotonin and noradrenaline. These are normally present in quite large quantities in the brain, and in particular in one set of structures.

The limbic system

The structures concerned are spread around various parts of the brain, but are linked in the form of a circuit called the **limbic system** (see Figure 1, overleaf).

The limbic system controls a lot of the body's processes, such as sleeping–waking cycles, temperature control, temper control, eating patterns and hormones; every hormone in the body is directly or indirectly under the control of the limbic system. It keeps all of these functions in balance with each other. The limbic system is essentially a giant thermostat or reverberating circuit, controlling many functions at once. Its most important function is to control mood.

It normally does this remarkably well. A human being's mood is usually very stable. For example, if you win a million pounds on the lottery, your mood does indeed rise, for a few days. It then returns to normal, with occasional peaks, mostly in the first few weeks, corresponding with buying your first Ferrari and the like. So mood isn't controlled consistently by events or the quality of your life, but by the limbic system.

But like every other system and structure in the body, it has a limit. If you bash a bone hard and consistently enough, it will break. So will the limbic system.

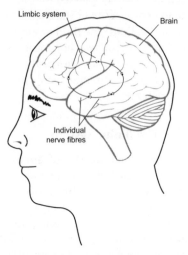

Figure 1 The limbic system (simplified)
This simplified diagram shows one chain of nerve fibres. The whole system consists of millions of such chains with complex inputs and outputs, which are not shown.

It can be caused to malfunction by a number of different factors. These include viral illnesses such as flu. Other precipitants of limbic system dysfunction are hormonal conditions, illicit drugs, too much alcohol, some prescribed medicines, too many major life changes, too many losses or facing choices involving conflicting needs. By far the commonest trigger, though, is stress.

The synapse

Whatever the cause, the end result is the same. If the limbic system is taken beyond its design limits, it will malfunction. The part of the limbic system that goes is the gap between the end of one nerve and the beginning of another, or the **synapse**, as shown in Figure 2. There are millions of these in the limbic system and they are the most vulnerable part of the circuit.

Transmitter chemicals, or neurotransmitters, are chemicals that transmit signals from one neuron or

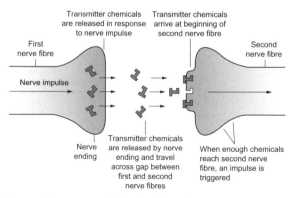

Figure 2 A synapse in the limbic system

nerve cell to another via the synapses, the site where the neurons meet. Transmitter chemicals include serotonin and noradrenaline, both believed to be implicated in the maintenance of mood. In clinical depression it is these transmitter chemicals that are affected. In response to stress or any of the other triggers listed above, the levels of these chemicals in the synapses of the limbic system plummet, and the limbic system grinds to a halt.

2

Symptoms

When the limbic system stops functioning, a characteristic set of symptoms arises. These symptoms are what define clinical depression and separate it out from other states, such as sadness, disgruntlement or stress. Most of these symptoms are under the heading of 'loss of'. It's pretty much a case of loss of everything – it is as if the whole body shuts down.

Cortisol

The symptom of feeling worse in the morning is a particular 'marker' for depressive illness and is caused by a hormonal change. Under normal circumstances the level of the hormone cortisol fluctuates through the day, with a high peak in the early morning and a gradual falling-off through the day until, by the evening, there is very little in circulation. However, in depressive illness, this morning peak is lost. Thus you feel worse in the morning. This is one demonstration, if there were any doubt, that depressive illness really is physical.

Who gets depressive illness?

One more important fact: depressive illness, or at least the commonest form, which is that caused by stress, nearly always happens to one type of

Symptoms in clinical depression

- Feeling worse in the morning and better as the day goes on.
- Loss of:
  - sleep (usually early morning waking)*
  - appetite*
  - energy
  - enthusiasm
  - concentration
  - memory**
  - confidence
  - self-esteem
  - sex drive
  - drive
  - enjoyment
  - patience
  - feelings
  - hope
  - love
  - and almost anything else you can think of.

* Both sleep and appetite can occasionally be increased, rather than decreased.
** Loss of memory is, in fact, apparent rather than real. What actually happens is that you can't concentrate during a depressive episode, so you don't take information in properly. Therefore the information isn't available later to recall.

person. He or she will have the following personality characteristics:

- (moral) strength
- reliability
- diligence
- a strong conscience
- a strong sense of responsibility

- a tendency to focus on the needs of others before one's own
- sensitivity
- vulnerability to criticism
- self-esteem dependent on the evaluation of others.

This person is the sort to whom you would turn if you had a problem to sort out upon which your life depended. She is a safe pair of hands and you can trust her with anything. Indeed, this person is usually admired, though often somewhat taken for granted by those around her. People are usually very surprised when she gets ill; indeed, she is the last person you would expect to have a breakdown.

But it isn't so surprising when you consider that depressive illness is a physical condition. Think about it: give a set of stresses to someone who is weak, cynical or lazy and he will quickly give up, so he will never get stressed enough to become ill. A strong person, on the other hand, will react to these pressures by trying to overcome them. So she keeps going, absorbing more and more, until, inevitably: BANG! The fuse blows.

That is what depression is: a blown fuse. Again, this isn't a metaphor. The limbic system is a type of fuse mechanism and when it blows, it doesn't matter how hard you try, you can't achieve anything. Once the fuse has blown, you can put 1,000 amps through it, but it won't do any good.

So turn the electricity off.

The point to hold on to now is that you are wrong in thinking you are weak and that you should be ashamed to have contracted this illness. *You have got it because you are too strong.*

What causes it?

I believe that a crucial part of beating the illness is knowing why you got it in the first place. Unfortunately, it's beyond the scope of this short book to cover this in detail, but do look up the pointers below in the full version of *Depressive Illness: The Curse of the Strong*, or perhaps note them for possible discussion in psychotherapy (see Chapter 7). In brief, here are some underlying reasons for depression.

- *Overactive superego*: an overcritical conscience formed early in life by harsh and judgemental parents.
- *Anger turned inward*: typically in someone whose needs are not met. Neglect leads to mounting frustration and, eventually, rage. This has to go somewhere, and, turned inward, can result in depressive symptoms.
- *Resonance with past loss*: for example, loss of a parent in childhood may not cause obvious depression at the time, but a significant loss in adult life – e.g. redundancy or bereavement – may resonate with an early loss that has been dormant for many years.
- *Maternal deprivation and attachment*: an adult who has not had her attachment needs met as a child will be overanxious and needy in relationships, causing her to meet with rejection and loss, leading to more anger, hopelessness and depression.

3

What to do when you get ill

Whatever your background and whichever route or routes you have taken into clinical depression, I invite you to consider the following:

You have done too much, been too strong and tried too hard for too long.

Now the fuse has blown. *It isn't your fault.* Far from it: you are worthy of praise and admiration, not the self-criticism you have been heaping on your own head for some time.

In order to achieve success that is worthwhile and wide-ranging, you must first learn to fail well.

Rest

But first you must give up the struggle. While you continue pushing yourself the body can't start to heal. It's a waste of time, anyway. You can't achieve much because your concentration, energy and judgement are at an all-time low. So stop. This means:

- taking time off work if this is at all possible;
- getting help at home with the kids and domestic chores;
- cancelling all those social events you have been dreading.

You are dreading them because you are well aware (your body is telling you) that *they will hurt you*. If you force yourself to endure them you will get worse. It also means:

- telling family, friends, your local charity and anyone else you do things for, that they are going to have to do without you for a while. If they complain, get them to read this book;
- above all, ignoring those who tell you to get more active and to pull yourself together, unless you want to be rude to them; that would be fine.

Coasting in neutral

The trouble is that if you just sit in a chair all day, you have far too much time to ruminate. Going to bed isn't the answer either. So there is a dilemma: how to stop yourself ruminating while not overusing your body's scant resources. In my experience, the average person in the pits of a depressive illness has no more than about 10–15 minutes of available energy for anything at all demanding before she gets tired. If she goes beyond this limit on a regular basis, she doesn't get better.

The answers are to find any way you can of keeping your brain just idling, to avoid any challenging activities wherever possible and to do what you have to in very small chunks.

Best of all, be passive. The ideal would be an undiluted diet of Australian soap operas, if you can stomach that sort of thing. They allow you to sit and not to ruminate – a sort of mental wallpaper, filling up the space and covering over the cracks.

Meanwhile, you can imitate a vegetable and allow your body to proceed with the task of healing. It will do this so long as you leave it alone to get on with it. If you can't cope with TV, then choose anything that you find easy to do. But beware: what you normally find easy may now be difficult. Take things as you find them now and avoid value judgements of the 'Oh, that's pathetic, I can't even . . .' type. Look for things that allow you to coast along in neutral.

Some don'ts

- Don't make any major life-altering decisions at this stage, especially ones that are potentially irrevocable. It's a bad idea for you to resign from your job at this stage, though this may well be a good idea later.
- Don't leave home.
- Don't sell anything.
- Don't cancel your holiday abroad yet. You may get better quicker than you think.
- And *don't harm yourself*. I know it seems hopeless now but it will all look very different in a little while when you get better.

Yes, you will get better. People recover from clinical depression. Don't punish yourself. Your feelings of guilt are a symptom of your illness and are very unlikely to be deserved. Yes, your illness may have affected your family, but *it isn't your fault*, any more than if you had developed pneumonia. So give yourself a break and let yourself be.

Your partner

Your spouse or partner may well be struggling with your illness. That is understandable; it is tough living with someone suffering from clinical depression, though not half as tough as having it yourself. You are victims of this misfortune together, with no one at fault. Try to show each other some compassion. Don't draw any conclusions about your impotence or loss of sex drive. It is down to the illness, and everything will come back to normal eventually, though it may take a while owing to the medication (see Chapter 4).

One of the worst symptoms, which makes you feel even more guilty, is loss of feelings for loved ones. Try not to worry; it will all come back. You haven't really lost your feelings; this is just a symptom.

4

Antidepressant medication

One of the most difficult parts of my job is often persuading patients who desperately need it to take antidepressant medication. The commonly cited reasons for declining are as follows:

'I prefer to do it on my own, without resorting to pills.' Why? Would you say the same if you had pneumonia? Choosing not to take antibiotics is risky and means you will remain ill for longer than you need to.

'Antidepressants aren't natural.' No they aren't, but what's your point? Naturally occurring substances are among the most toxic drugs in our pharmacopoeia; warfarin, for example, is used to treat blood clots but is also the active ingredient in rat poison. Forget the idea that natural is best; it's bunkum.

'Antidepressants are addictive.' No they aren't. You can become reliant on them if you take them for too long, but that is true of anything and doesn't mean the same as addiction. Occasionally, people who stop their medication abruptly can get withdrawal symptoms, but that just means you should stop your medication as advised by your doctor, in a gradual manner. Very few people have problems on withdrawal if they do this.

'Antidepressants give you a false high and change your personality.' No they don't. At best an antidepressant can bring the level of the transmitter chemicals in your limbic system and your mood back to *normal* (see Figure 3, p. 16). Forget anything you've read saying you can use Prozac as a party drug; you can't.

'I've read that Prozac can make you violent.' Forget lurid newspaper articles suggesting it turns people into psychopaths who go around chopping up their families. Oh, give me a break! Look, Prozac is an ordinary antidepressant; quite a good one for some people, but it isn't a wonder drug and it isn't a devil's potion. Newspapers dream up sensations to sell papers and, having talked to friends and colleagues from around the world, I have no doubt that the UK press is the worst and most cynical in the civilized world. Beware the press.

Having said this, Prozac, like the other drugs in its class (the SSRIs – see page 20) can make some people feel worse for the first 10 days or so, with an increase in anxiety and agitation. It is possible that some reports of violence in people taking these drugs may relate to this fairly uncommon side effect. If you feel very agitated when you start the drug, get in touch with your doctor and if necessary, stop taking it.

'I tried an antidepressant for a few days before and it made me feel worse.' That's because you didn't take it for long enough. Side effects are at their worst in the first couple of weeks of treatment, then generally fade away (though a few may persist). The beneficial effects don't usually start until around two weeks into treatment and it may take six weeks or longer for the full benefits of the drug to be felt. Try again and, this time, persist if you can. If the side effects are too bad, go back to your doctor and tell her. She will change you to a different type of drug with which you will probably have a much better time.

'I've tried one for several weeks before and it didn't work.' OK, you've given it a fair try, but it may have needed an increase in dosage. Around 50 per cent of people who respond to an antidepressant need an increase in the starting dose a few weeks into treatment. Again, go back to your doctor.

'I looked at the patient information leaflet (PIL) that came with my tablets and the list of side effects scared me so much that I decided not to take them.' These leaflets are the bane of my life. I'll bet it was a politician who decided on them. Like the other political 'improvements' to the health service, they have done untold harm. The PIL has to list every significant side effect that has been described anywhere in the world, even once. You're about as likely to suffer from some of them as you are to win the National Lottery. Medications are pretty safe if you take them sensibly; certainly a lot safer than leaving your illness untreated.

How antidepressants work

Antidepressants work by bringing the levels of the transmitter chemicals back to normal and making the nerves more sensitive, so that the limbic system starts running again (see Figure 3, overleaf). There are several different antidepressant medications. They are all effective in the majority of people suffering from clinical depression, around 60–70 per cent responding well to any one medication, but each drug covers a slightly different 60–70 per cent. If you're unlucky, you may need to go through a few different types to find the one that does it for you. The chances are that the first drug you go on will work, so long as you take it for long enough. Remember that side effects are at

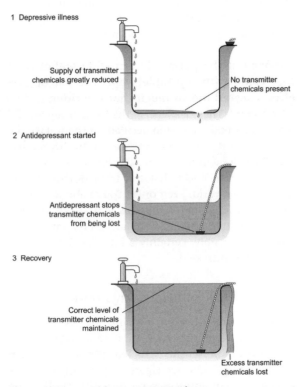

Figure 3 How antidepressants work

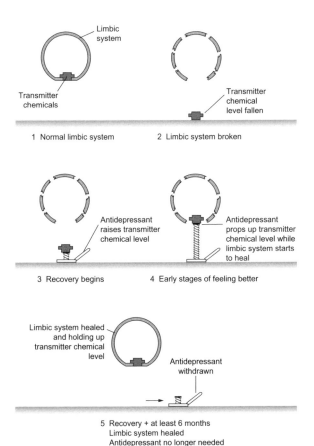

Figure 4 Keeping antidepressants going for long enough: a schematic representation

their worst in the first week or two, while the beneficial effects usually take a few weeks to kick in.

It is crucial that you keep taking the medication once you get well. Patients sometimes stop taking the drug as soon as they feel well. As often as not, they relapse, then lose faith in medication. No, the reason for the return of symptoms was that the limbic system hadn't yet had time to heal. That takes weeks to months.

We usually advise continuing the antidepressant for *at least six months from the point when you start feeling well* (see Figure 4, p. 17). If you stop it as soon as you feel well, you've got roughly a 60 per cent chance of relapse in the following few weeks (see Figure 5); poor odds. Another month and the risk is in the region of 35 per cent, at three months 20–25 per cent; still too high. At six months it is around 15 per cent, at a year 10 per cent and at two years still 10 per cent.

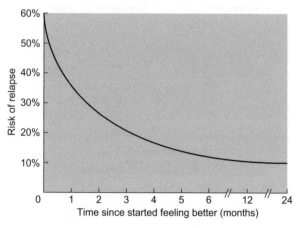

Figure 5 Risk of relapse decreases with longer duration of treatment

Remember, though, that the clock doesn't even start until you begin feeling well. Your doctor will advise you on this.

Also, please remember: *don't stop your medication abruptly*. Withdraw it over several weeks under the direction of your doctor.

Types of antidepressant

The following are the main classes of antidepressants.

Tricyclics

These were the first antidepressants to be used, back in the 1950s. They worked and are still used today. Indeed, at high enough doses, they are at least as effective as any of the modern drugs. One problem, though, is that at these doses they can have quite a few side effects. Most of them are sedative, and they can also cause weight gain.

The biggest problem with these drugs is that they are exceptionally dangerous in overdosage. Sadly, over-dosage is something that sometimes happens in people who are severely ill with clinical depression. Having said that, I do sometimes prescribe tricyclics, as they often work in the minority of cases when the modern drugs fail.

If you do take a tricyclic antidepressant, please take it at the dosage prescribed; they don't work if you take them at too low a dose, or erratically.

Monoamine oxidase inhibitors (MAOIs)

These drugs, or at least the original ones, aren't often used nowadays. They are rather inconvenient to take owing to the extensive food restrictions. These include cheese, yeast products (including beer), red wine (particularly Chianti), and any meat that isn't fresh. You have to take these restrictions seriously; ignoring them could, at worst, lead to a stroke. There are quite a few interactions with other medicines too. You need to tell your pharmacist that you're on them before you take any over-the-counter medicines.

Selective serotonin reuptake inhibitors (SSRIs)

These drugs are a lot safer and easier to take. As their group name suggests, they work on just one of the two chemicals involved in clinical depression, serotonin. Some examples are fluoxetine (Prozac), paroxetine (Seroxat), sertraline (Lustral) and citalopram (Cipramil).

The SSRIs aren't without their problems, but side effects are usually transient and manageable. These mostly occur in the first couple of weeks of treatment, and include some nausea and/or headache. A small number of patients, maybe 10 per cent, suffer distressing agitation, though this also doesn't last. In fact, though, the National Institute of Health and Care Excellence (NICE) has taken this side effect very seriously indeed and has advised against the use of SSRIs in adolescents, warning of the potential for an increase in suicide risk and violence in the early stages of taking the drug. Of course, if you experience very severe agitation early on in treatment, this could put you at increased risk, and if necessary you may need to stop taking the drug and consult your doctor. However, most people get nothing very much at all in the way of adverse side effects from SSRIs.

Except, that is, sexual dysfunction. At least 50 per cent of my patients get this to a greater or lesser degree and it may last for as long as you take the tablets (plus a short period while the drug gets out of your system). It's not you, it's the tablets, and some other antidepressants can do the same thing.

Other new-generation antidepressants

Since the advent of the SSRIs, a number of further drugs have become available. These reflect the fact that some people don't recover with a drug working on the serotonin system alone.

While the other transmitter chemical, noradrenaline, usually rises automatically when the levels of serotonin come back to normal, this doesn't always occur. Sometimes the noradrenaline system needs to be tweaked more directly. These drugs fit the bill.

Mood stabilizers

These are drugs normally only used for people who are prone to recurrent episodes of depression.

The first mood stabilizer to be discovered, lithium carbonate, is a naturally occurring salt. It's the most frequently effective, though just how effective in stress-induced depression isn't clear yet. Lithium is inconvenient to take, mainly because it requires regular blood tests. Without these, there would be a small, but significant, risk to your kidneys. Lithium also occasionally affects the thyroid gland.

The other mood stabilizers require less frequent monitoring, but have a rather lower success rate. They are drugs primarily used to control epilepsy.

Herbal preparations

I'm not going to go into these in detail here; I believe the rationale for preferring them to be bogus. St John's

Wort is effective in some cases. Many people seem to tolerate it well, but it probably isn't as good in severe clinical depression as the medicines listed above. It does have some interactions with other drugs. Yes, it is a drug. It works on the same chemical systems as other antidepressants. However, there isn't sufficient evidence available on any other herbal preparation advertised as treating depression for me to give it to my dog, let alone recommend it to you, my reader.

A word about electroconvulsive therapy (ECT)

Most psychiatrists still use ECT, but only rarely, *in extremis*. I only suggest it if my patient is at risk of serious harm because he has stopped eating and/or drinking, if all other available treatments have failed (it takes a long time to try them all), or if, subjectively, the torment of his illness is so dreadful that a compassionate human being cannot leave him in his hell-hole for a day longer than necessary. In these cases, it can be a life-saver. And, if you talk to people who have had it, it isn't a distressing experience, any more than any anaesthetic is.

5

Recovery

There you are, I told you that you would start to feel better eventually. Sometimes it happens quickly and sometimes it takes longer, with one or more changes of treatment along the way. But, in the vast majority, it happens.

Now, this is where it gets a bit complicated. Recovery isn't, unless you are very lucky, a smooth path upward. If you try to hurry yourself to full recovery, the process can be very turbulent indeed and take an age. If you do everything right, there are still usually a lot of ups and downs along the way, but they are minimized. Assuming you follow my advice, you can expect a pattern of recovery something like that shown in Figure 6.

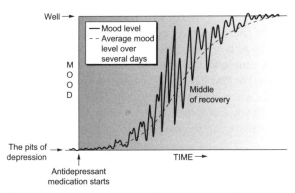

Figure 6 Graph of recovery of mood versus time

As you can see from the graph, it takes a while for anything to happen after you start taking the anti-depressant. Then you get the odd slightly better day. But not much and not often; most days are still a torment. As time goes on, though, the fluctuations get larger, until, in the middle of recovery, the swings day to day are enormous. One day you feel almost back to normal, then the next you feel as bad as ever.

Suicidal thoughts – DON'T ACT

A sad fact is that the commonest time for a person to take his life is not when he is in the pits of depression, but at this point, when he is beginning to get better. One reason for this is that, when you have had a really good day, the bad day that follows is thrown into sharp relief and so seems even worse than the gloom of the days when every day was bad. The other is that, if you happen to be someone for whom energy and volition come back before mood improves, there is a risk of your getting the wherewithal to carry through self-destructive thoughts that you have had for some time, but not had the energy to act upon.

The crucial message at this time is: *don't act. You are going to be better soon; this is only a bad day.*

As time goes on the fluctuations in mood again lessen. The bad days get less bad, less frequent, shorter than a whole day, and eventually peter out altogether, though you can sometimes be surprised by a rotten one quite late in the process.

Don't overdo it

It is crucial not to overreact to these fluctuations. Instead, enjoy the good days, but be careful not to overdo it. On the bad days, just accept them and wait for tomorrow in the knowledge that further good days will come with ever-increasing frequency as time goes on.

So how much can you do at any particular point in the recovery process? The truth is, I haven't the faintest idea, but you do *because your body tells you.*

- If you overdo it physically, your body starts feeling heavy and lethargic, as if wading through treacle.
- If you overdo it mentally, you start not being able to think straight and you can read the same page of a book three times without being aware of a word that was written.
- If you overdo it socially, you will have spoken to someone for five minutes without knowing what subject is being discussed.

If you keep going past the point of these warning signs, you will, sure as eggs is eggs, have a rotten day tomorrow. If you repeatedly do so, you will experience the yo-yo effect. On good days, fired up by enthusiasm, you determine to catch up on all those tasks you have been unable to complete through the illness. You ignore the cues your body gives you after ten minutes telling you that you are tired and should stop. So you carry on, through the barrier of tiredness.

From this moment, you have condemned yourself to a rotten 36 hours (or up to 72 hours if you overdo it grossly). Your body goes back into shut-down, forcing you to rest the next day (or three). This is all that is needed for healing to resume, so you then have another good day, which you use to rush around again. Another bad day follows and so on, and on and on.

If you do it this way, recovery can take an age.

Much better to do what your body tells you. You will get better quickest if you listen to what it says. It gives you all the data you need. Yes, I know this can be very difficult in the real world, with a family to look after and a mortgage to pay, but it is in everybody's interests for you to take it slowly at this point. Someone else will have to help with chores such as the shopping and taking the kids to school.

They would if you had a broken leg – ironic, as depressive illness (or a fracture of the limbic system) is a much more serious condition than a broken leg. So just in case you or those around you haven't got the message yet, let me say it, loud and clear, one more time: *clinical depression is a physical illness and you have to take it seriously.*

The Hoover in the middle of the room

So how do you start becoming more active once recovery begins? The answer is that you start by doing bits of things. An indication of whether you are getting this stage right I call 'the Hoover in the middle of the room test'. If I were to come into your house in the early stages of your recovery, I should see a whole set of part-done tasks and the Hoover sitting in the middle of the sitting-room floor.

If you have a good day you might feel you would like to do a bit of spring cleaning. So you get the Hoover out. Halfway through hoovering, after 15 minutes, you start feeling heavy, tired and lethargic. Now, this is the crucial moment: you *switch off the Hoover and leave it standing in the middle of the sitting-room floor.* You go off for an hour and sit down, watch the television, potter around, or whatever. When you feel your energy coming back, you can do a bit more, but only until you feel tired again, at which point you again stop. By the end of the day you may have done about half the house. Because you have stayed within your body's limits, you may well feel all right the next day and be able to finish the task; if not, then the day after that.

So don't push yourself; ease yourself towards recovery at a pace your body can manage. If you do this you will find that gradually, with some hiccups, you will be able to do more and more.

Use your common sense and listen to the messages your body is giving you. They are true. Take your recovery as it is, rather than how you would have it be. You'll be well soon enough; just let it happen.

6

Staying well

If you look at most textbooks on depressive illness, you will read that it is usually a recurrent condition. That is, most people who get an episode go on to have one or more further episodes in the future. I don't find this to be so. While some people do have recurrent spells of depression, they are in two groups. The first group comprises those who have a recurrent illness that is independent of, and largely unaffected by, stress. I am not dealing with people who have this type of condition here. The second group, which is much the larger, comprises those who get further episodes of clinical depression because they have learnt and changed nothing from their first episode.

The bottom line is this. *Antidepressants and rest can get you better, but if nothing changes it's a matter of time before you get ill again.* If you can change the way you operate, so that you experience balanced give and take in your life rather than just being a tool for others to use, there is no need to get a further episode of depressive illness. If you can't, you probably need some form of psychotherapy (see Chapter 7).

> *If you keep putting 13 amps through a 5 amp fuse, it will keep blowing.*

Once you have recovered from an episode of depressive illness, it is possible not only to stay well but also to become happier than you have been for years. In order to achieve this, though, you must understand why you became ill in the first place and then make the necessary changes to put these circumstances right. You must make choices in your life.

All change

There are lots of apparently valid reasons not to make the changes you need. When I urge a busy businessperson to look at the choices in his life, I tend to get a scornful response: 'Choices, what choices? When you have responsibilities, you have no option but to soldier on; the school fees and the mortgage have to be paid.' But he is wrong. There are changes you can make to your life without changing the children's schools or moving house. These changes won't be easy and will involve learning to say no, and to be more assertive in setting out your needs.

Make choices for yourself and take the opportunities that are presented to you. Some of those around you will grumble; you need to keep an eye on them – they are the takers. They will turn on you when you can't do it for them any more, and won't be there for you in your hour of need. Those friends who really care for you will welcome your taking more for yourself. In any case, you need to take responsibility for your own happiness. Don't expect others to make you happy; forge it yourself. If your family are struggling because they have got used to you doing everything for them, understand their distress but leave it to them to work through it. It's their struggle, not yours.

Make the most of crisis

This turning of the worm may create a crisis. The ancient Greeks knew this issue well. The word 'crisis' comes from the Greek, meaning literally 'a time of opportunity'. Miss the opportunity to destabilize the system you are in now and you condemn yourself to more of what you've had for years. *If nothing changes, everything remains the same.*

This time of turmoil is when things can change, if you choose for them to do so. But you are the one who will have to do it. Nobody else will; they have become too comfortable with the status quo. Why should they change things when there has always been you to rely on?

Guilt is good

Changing things in your favour will make you feel guilty. That's a problem that stops many of my patients in their tracks and prevents them from creating enduring change in their lives.

Well, my friends, I've got news for you: *guilt is good*. In fact it is essential. If a newly recovered patient of mine tells me she is feeling guilty about the changes she is making and the demands she is putting on to others, I go 'Hurrah!' That means she is making the changes she needs to, in order to forge a life for herself that is sustainable and capable of producing happiness in the long run (for herself and those around her). But if guilt is good, resentment is bad. If you find yourself feeling resentment, you are not making the changes you need to or sufficiently asserting yourself.

Imagine depression as a dark room: there is only one way out to the bright garden of health and happiness – and that is through a doorway marked 'Guilt'.

Finding the middle ground

Having said this, beware of swinging to extremes (see Figure 7). In British culture we have a tendency to do this. Occasionally I see an unassertive, down-trodden spouse swing to become a demanding and aggressive tyrant. Mr Dependable starts having affairs and getting drunk. On the surface, these massive changes seem inexplicable, but they are not. In fact, little has changed, because opposites are very similar. Unassertiveness and aggressiveness are two sides of the same coin, as are extremes of diligence and laziness, or reliable self-denial and impulsive hedonism. The really radical change is the middle ground, or balance. It is

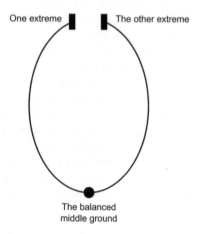

One extreme ∎   ∎ The other extreme

The balanced
middle ground

Figure 7 The radical centre

this that you need in order to avoid oscillating from one extreme to another, without enduring change.

I'm not advocating mediocrity here, just sustainability. The key to performing well in the long term without blowing a fuse is *operating at just below peak capacity*. There is a graph that demonstrates this called the Yerke–Dodson curve (see Figure 8).

This is a graph of level of performance against level of arousal. I use the term arousal because it implies a scale from very low to very high, but you could just as well call it anxiety, tension, alertness, excitement or stress. They are all different aspects of the same thing. At zero arousal you are asleep, so you can't do

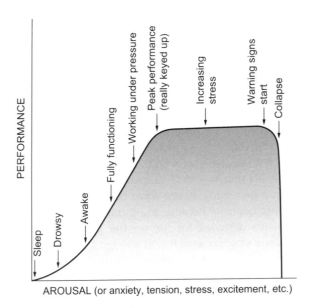

AROUSAL (or anxiety, tension, stress, excitement, etc.)

Figure 8 The Yerke–Dodson curve

anything. To work effectively in a competitive environment you must be quite aroused. A bit more and you're at your peak – really keyed up, flying, ready for anything. The trouble is, this level is a greasy pole. You either keep going up, or you slide down. The most efficient way of operating is to be just below the peak, rising to this level for brief spells as you need to. If you try to stay at your peak, you will gradually slide upward, to an increasingly high level of arousal, when you are beginning to feel the strain.

As Figure 8 shows, there is quite a bit of a plateau, but when the fall-off happens there isn't much warning. Your arousal level goes up and up and up, then – wallop! You fall over the edge and you can't function at all.

The first time this happens it may take the form of 'losing it': irrational behaviour, running around like a headless chicken or exploding at someone. Collapse may exhibit as a panic attack, in which you feel extreme fear, breathlessness, palpitations, sweating, light-headedness and a feeling of being separated from the world by a thick pane of glass.

If you get a panic attack, unpleasant though it is, don't panic! It's a normal reaction. Though you may feel as if you're going to have a heart attack and die, take it from me: you won't. The problem isn't your heart, it's that you've been running so hot that your brain is perceiving danger when there isn't any.

This happens because the human body is out of date. It's designed for life on the primordial plain millions of years ago. If you emerge from your cave to be confronted by a sabre-toothed tiger, you're going to have to react very quickly or you die. Your body, with the aid of the hormone adrenaline, gears up for explosive action with lightning speed. Within a couple of heartbeats your muscles are in a state of tension, your heart is pumping faster, you are breathing rapidly, your nerves are all super-sensitive, your senses are hyper-acute and you will experience problems 'at both ends' (to make you as light as possible, so you can run a bit faster – even a kilogram may be the difference between life and death).

Several of my patients – who, as you can imagine, the illness being what it is, include many of the good and the great – tell me that *you can achieve 99 per cent of the output with 60 per cent of the effort.* And it will be sustainable.

Pointless activity

In my view it is also important to spend some of your time in pointless activity. If you are all the time doing things that bring tangible results, the chances are that you are running too hot. Why do you have to be useful all the time anyway? What are you trying to prove, and to whom? Try making yourself stop, for some time every day and for a longer period at weekends. That's why I play golf. It's difficult, time consuming and completely pointless. I'm not very good and I love it! Being allowed to do something really badly without anybody being upset is a joy.

Keep it simple: three questions

I like to keep it simple. There are just three questions that separate out those of my patients who stay well after recovery from those who fit the description given on pp. 5–7 and continue to experience episodes of illness. They are these:

1 *What is it all for?*
2 *What do I want?*
3 *Where is the balance in my life?*

If these questions sound like ancient Greek to you, you've got a problem; it's a matter of time before you become ill again. If you can answer them, you've got every chance of remaining healthy and, in due course, becoming happier than you've been in a long time.

Work out your own answers. Then put them past your best friend (not your spouse). If you get them right, congratulations! You've just won health and, if you're lucky, happiness.

You won't always be happy, of course, because sometimes life throws you some unpleasant ordeals. When it does, be sad. Don't put on a brave face. But be flexible. In the storm, the stout oak falls, but the bendy reed survives. *Be bendy.*

7

Psychotherapy

Most people don't need long-term exploratory psychotherapy. Considering the models in this book and working on the implications they contain may well be enough. If you can answer the three questions I posed on page 36, and if you can change the way you run your life based on those answers, you don't need psychotherapy. You can probably look forward to a happier and healthier life. You will look back on this episode of depressive illness as a blessing, the pivotal point when your life turned around for the better.

But it may not be as easy as that. You may find yourself compelled to keep overloading, neglecting and abusing yourself for reasons you can't fathom. Then you need psychotherapy of one kind or another. There are four forms of therapy that will probably be fairly accessible locally under the NHS.

1 *Supportive counselling* is not seeking to explore any background or make any very profound changes, beyond those necessary to allow you time and space to heal. It seeks to build up your defences against the problems surrounding you, by talking things through. Most members of the community mental health team can do this work and counsellors are available in many general practice surgeries.

2 *Group psychotherapy* comes in different forms. Most psychiatric day hospitals and community mental health resource centres have a range of available

group activities, all the way from simple relaxation training to fully fledged cognitive therapy or sometimes even exploratory psychotherapy. Many people are naturally reluctant to share their problems in public, but if any group sessions are recommended to you, consider them seriously. You are likely to find a lot of wisdom, practical advice and skills to help you cope, and people who think like you, in these groups.

3 *Short-term focal therapy* does exactly what it says on the tin. It doesn't seek to dig into the past, except in order to understand your present conflicts and why these stresses are making you ill now. It seeks solutions to your present problems, rather than working through a lot of issues from the past. It usually involves a session with a therapist once a week, or fortnight, for a few months.

4 *Cognitive therapy* looks, here and now, at the way you think and tries to change your negative and self-defeating thinking patterns through challenging them.

Individual psychodynamic psychotherapy/grieving

Psychodynamic psychotherapy is a more in-depth form of psychotherapy that seeks to identify the driving (or psychodynamic) issues in your life. Although available in theory on the NHS, it is probably best sought privately from a reputable therapist.

Identifying the root of your problems does not make them go away. Having found those issues throughout your life that you didn't deal with at the time, you need now to *work them through*. This process is easiest to understand with reference to a phenomenon that I specifically don't deal with in this book: grieving.

Most people know that, if you lose a loved one, you have to grieve. If you don't do so at the time, the grief will drip away through your life in the decades that follow. Grieving, painful though it is, allows you, in due course, to move on. It isn't ever OK; of course it isn't. But you are able to be *free*. Free to experience the whole range of human emotions, rather than just sadness; to be sad sometimes, desolate occasionally, and at other times, unexpectedly, to experience pleasure, and even joy. If you are experiencing grief right now, you won't believe this to be possible; the

Acting out

Your role in therapy is important. In my view the single most important determinant in the success or failure of psychotherapy is the degree of **acting out**. This refers to *acting* on your feelings and emotions *outside* the therapy sessions. The opposite is **talking** or **working in therapy**. If you act out your issues, nothing ever changes because there is no emotion left for the work of therapy. And it is emotion that is the fuel of therapy.

The commonest form of acting out that I see in my patients is excessive caring. There are times when, as I tell my patient to forge more time and space for herself, I know she won't do so; I can see it in her eyes. She is spending her life running away from guilt, having traded her guilt for a lorry-load of exhaustion and quiet, resigned resentment. Therapy doesn't work, because she is too busy rushing around tending to folks for it to take hold. Soon enough she drops therapy as she hasn't got time for it.

If she's you, then I'm sorry, but you're choosing illness. Recognize what you're doing and take responsibility for it. When you're ready, make a different choice.

mere suggestion is probably slightly offensive. But feel, without pushing your feelings away, and, mark my words, it will happen.

This is working through – the working through of a terrible loss. The process of psychotherapy does the same thing. You are being taken through a grieving process, in a way, for what should have been. In the same way that someone emerges from grief if he faces it, you emerge from psychotherapy more healthy by working through those issues that you didn't deal with at the time.

Cognitive behavioural therapy (CBT)

Cognitive behavioural therapy, in the hands of a skilled therapist, is beautifully simple. It simply invites you to look at the truth accurately, rather than in your usual selectively negative fashion. CBT usually involves a considerable amount of homework and its success depends on you doing the work properly.

While you would have thought that the sort of person who gets clinical depression would be sure to pursue this task with diligence, this isn't always the case. There are several reasons for this.

First, the treatment is often started too soon. In the pits of depression, you can't make a cup of tea, let alone keep a complex diary of thoughts and alternative self-statements. In my view, cognitive therapy is, in any case, better at *keeping* you well than *getting* you well, so there's no enormous hurry to get it started. There is always a bit of a conflict between the need for rest in early recovery and the need of the therapy for homework. You'll just have to make your own judgements on this as you go along. Concentrate more on resting early on, but more on the therapy once you are quite a bit better.

Second, you tend to think of yourself as bottom of

the list of priorities. By the time you have kept everyone else happy, you've already overdone it and so have no time or energy left for working at the therapy.

Third, there is a part of you that is self-destructive (I mention 'Overactive superego', 'Anger turned inward', page 8). This part will tend to have you subconsciously sabotage the treatment, by passively resisting the therapist's efforts. I can testify how frustrating this is. But, if you can become conscious of this tendency, you have real choice. You could choose to overrule your self-destructive tendency and, against your instincts, do the work you need to do.

Fourth and finally, the exact same thought patterns that underpin depression will tend to dissuade you from working on yourself and your needs. 'Oh, what's the point, it won't work, nothing ever does. In any case, I can't do anything about my life.'

Look, forget your judgements about whether or not things will change. It doesn't matter much whether or not you believe in the therapy, whether you enjoy it or whether you want to do it. *Just do it*. The point of it will emerge later.

If you do the work in between the sessions that your therapist asks of you, there is an excellent chance of success. Cognitive therapy has a proven track record. From my observation, there is a fair chance of achieving the changes that you need to in between six and twenty sessions. After that, it's down to you. Cognitive therapy only works if your changed way of thinking leads to *a change in the way you operate*.

Make use of your new thinking

So, now use your more accurate thinking to make some choices in your life. The disaster that you always assumed would follow doing what you want and making a shift in your own favour, probably won't. You're now beginning to realize that and to see the exciting possibilities that it brings. Grab the opportunity. Some people will be unhappy about these changes, though not your real friends. In any case, it is their responsibility to adapt to the new order of things, not yours to organize it for them. This isn't belligerence, it is common sense.

Check your language

It's worth checking, from time to time, that you aren't slipping back into old ways. You can do this by noting the language you use. If you frequently use the words in the left-hand column, you need to do some more work on your thinking. If those in the right-hand column turn up more often, you'll probably achieve health and happiness.

Illness words	*Wellness words*
Must	Want
Have to	Choose
Fail	Learn
100%	Balance
Can't	Can
Resentment	Responsibility
What if	Opportunity

8

Some skills for problem areas

As we have seen, people who get stress-induced depressive illness tend to run too hot. They spend too much of their lives putting in too much effort. When confronted by a sea of troubles, they try to deal with them all at once. By now this will be a familiar picture. When they get overwhelmed they just push harder. Because they are so overaroused, they have difficulty in getting to sleep and then, when they become ill, they start waking in the early hours of the morning as well. Then they deal with the mounting tiredness by trying to push their way through it. So the conditions are in place for the fuse to blow.

Part of the solution, as I have outlined, is to change the way you operate, so you

- take on less and
- reserve more time and space for yourself.

The other part is to learn some skills that allow you to run at a lower level of arousal. This will help you feel less anxious and make it easier to sleep well.

Relaxation

The best way to combat stress is to learn and become expert at a relaxation exercise. There are several relaxation tapes available, and videos on YouTube. Some people benefit from yoga techniques learnt in a group

A relaxation exercise

Spend 15–20 minutes on this exercise.

1 Find a suitable place to relax. A bed or an easy chair is ideal, but anywhere will do, preferably somewhere quiet and private. If your seat in the office or a house full of children is all there is, it can still be done.
2 Try to clear your mind of thoughts as far as you can.
3 Take three very slow, very deep breaths (10–15 seconds to breathe in and out once).
4 Imagine a neutral figure. An example might be the number 1. Don't choose any object or figure with an emotional significance, such as a ring or a person, for example. Let it fill your mind. See it in your mind's eye, give it a colour, try to see it in 3D and repeat it to yourself, under your breath, many times over. Continue until it fills your mind.
5 Slowly change to imagine yourself somewhere quiet, peaceful and pleasurable. This may be a favourite place or situation, or a pleasant scene from your past. Be there, and notice all the feelings, in each sense. See it, feel it, hear it and smell it. Spend some time there.
6 Slowly change to be aware of your body. Notice any tension in your body. Take each group of muscles in turn, and tense, then relax them two or three times each. Include fingers, hands, arms, shoulders, neck, face, chest, tummy, buttocks, thighs, legs, feet and toes. Be aware of the feeling of relaxation. When the process is complete, spend some time in this relaxed state.
7 Slowly get up and go about your business.

Don't hurry this procedure, and remember to practise. It will work.

setting. Some find that following a written set of instructions helps them better, by allowing them to do the exercise at their own pace with their own mental imagery. What follows is just one example of such a technique, but one that many of my patients have found helpful.

Whichever way you choose, the essential point is that it needs a lot of practice. Persevere, because when you really master the technique you will find that it changes your life, allowing you to deal with situations that previously you could not have coped with at all. The people who benefit most from relaxation exercises are those who put them top of their list of priorities and practise for at least half an hour every day, come hell or high water.

Problem-solving

The principle of problem-solving is simple: take a set of problems or one big problem and split it up into smaller pieces. Let's take an example. You are in a financial mess. This problem is too big to manage as a whole, so split it up:

1 I'm above my overdraft limit at the bank.
2 My creditors are getting insistent.
3 I'm spending beyond my means.
4 My debtors aren't paying up.
5 The mortgage rate has gone up.
6 The car is on its last legs.
7 Christmas is just around the corner.

Now you have a set of smaller and more manageable problems to sort out. Take each one in turn and 'brainstorm' some possible actions. This means including all your ideas on what to do, the apparently bad ones as well as the obviously sensible ones. For example, for problem 1 a possible list might be:

(a) Ask the manager to extend my overdraft limit.
(b) Explain that the problem is largely of cash flow, that I am addressing it and it should only be temporary.
(c) Take out a short-term loan.
(d) Borrow from friends/relatives.
(e) Cut out items of expenditure (see Problem 3).
(f) Ignore it.
(g) Do more overtime.
(h) Move house.
(i) Change job.

Now think each option through and reject those that don't work. Talk it through with someone, if it helps.

Of course, following this structure for dealing with problems does not make them go away, but it does give you more control over them. Stress tends to happen when you feel that you have lost control over your life. You can't get the control back through effort alone. You need to act strategically, with organization and patience. Don't try to make it all happen at once.

Time management

If you find yourself harassed and overburdened, I would strongly recommend that you draw up a weekly time plan (Figure 9), with spaces for unforeseen events and for rest. This works even for the most irregular of lifestyles, such as bringing up children.

	Monday	Tuesday	Wednesday	Thursday	Friday	Saturday	Sunday
9 a.m.		spare for crises and problems		filing	deliver report	shopping	
10 a.m.	admin meeting		personal work	computer work	travel		
11 a.m.					meet with client		
Noon				prepare reports			
1 p.m.		L	U N	C H			rest
2 p.m.	personal work	travelling	presentation	meeting about report	travel personal work	rest	
3 p.m.		meeting	rest				
4 p.m.			travelling	admin	prepare next week's time plan		
5 p.m.							
Evening	rest	prepare presentation	late meeting	going out	rest	theatre	

Figure 9 A weekly time plan

Thought-stopping

When you are stressed you often find that a thought
sticks in your mind and you can't get rid of it, which
makes you even more tense. The following technique,
again with practice, can help you to clear your mind so
that you can get on with what you are doing or think
about something else.

- When you are alone, suddenly make a loud noise.
  Remember the sudden sensation.
- When you find yourself mulling over repetitive
  thoughts, bring this memory into your mind. Allow
  it to give you a jolt.
- Say sharply to yourself: 'Stop!' This does not have to
  be out loud, but imagine yourself saying it sharply
  and loudly.
- Substitute another thought that is relevant and realistic in your situation, or go and do something that
  requires concentration.

Sleep tips

Depressive illness wrecks your sleep. Usually your sleep pattern will return to normal once recovery has occurred, but sometimes poor sleep, resulting from running too hot, predates the illness. There are ways of sleeping better without sleeping tablets.

Catnaps and siestas

Your sleep requirement is calculated as a total over 24 hours. If you sleep for a couple of hours during the day, the total sleep you can expect the next night will fall by two hours. The loss usually occurs in the first half of the night, so it feels as if you can't get to sleep at the time that you feel you should. In fact, your usual 11 p.m. has just been delayed to around 1 a.m. If you get upset about this, sleep may be delayed further.

Coping with short-term sleep loss

In several studies, subjects were deprived of a night's sleep and then tested on a range of mental and manual skills. On most tests there wasn't a lot of difference between their performance and that of subjects who had been given a full night's sleep, but because the test results were of no concern to them they hadn't worried about their sleep loss. The best advice is as follows:

- Have a regular time to go to bed and stick to it.
- If you can't sleep on one particular night, don't worry.
- Instead, practise a relaxation exercise (see page 44). Effective relaxation confers many of the restorative benefits of sleep and will allow you to be fighting fit the next day, whether you sleep well or not.
- Above all, *don't use alcohol to help you sleep.* It will make things worse.

Tea and coffee

Most Britons drink a lot of coffee and/or tea. Both contain caffeine. If you have difficulty sleeping, it is wise to have your last cup before 6 p.m. Also, look out for some soft drinks. Many contain caffeine in considerable amounts.

A hot milky drink

The manufacturers of drinking chocolate and other such beverages have long extolled their virtues to assist good sleep. Most of us treat this claim sceptically, but in fact it is based on sound scientific fact. The benefits of these drinks can mostly be gained by a cup of hot milk, but drinking chocolate tastes better.

Exercise

The body uses sleep as a way of recuperating after the physical (and mental) rigours of the day. If there haven't been any rigours, sleep is deemed unnecessary. To sleep soundly, it is wise to take some exercise every day. Jumping in and out of the car and raising the glass to your lips don't count. Regular exercise (taken sensibly, according to your level of fitness) is, of course, good for your health anyway, and there is increasing evidence that it helps combat stress and improve your mood.

Of course, this only applies when you are well (even if stressed). Exercise is protective against developing clinical depression, but in the depths of the illness, in any more than very small bursts, makes it worse and delays recovery. So if you are suffering from depression, hold your horses; wait until you have recovered, then get as fit as you like.

Heat and ventilation

Being very hot or cold inhibits sleep, as does a stuffy atmosphere. It is surprising how high the carbon dioxide concentration can get in a room with windows and door closed and two people sleeping in it. This stale air tends to retard falling asleep and cause interruptions in the pattern of sleep through the night.

Meals

Eating at regular times helps to develop a pattern that the body clock can follow. Of course, this isn't always possible if you have a job with irregular hours or are looking after a baby, but the nearer you can get to a regular pattern of eating times, the better your sleep is likely to be. The same applies to other aspects of your life. An uncertain lifestyle without any routine does not encourage the body to develop the rhythms that lead to a regular sleep–wake cycle. It is important, as far as possible, to go to bed at roughly the same time most evenings and to retire neither hungry nor overfull.

Books, TV and so on

It is unfortunate that the TV companies tend to put on horror films and cops-and-robbers shows late at night. Watching such programmes can seriously damage your sleep because, whatever their quality, they are arousing, with lots of death and destruction. Another annoying thing that I have noticed is that late-night television announcers (and weather forecasters) talk to you as if you were a two-year-old child. This high-pitched smiling patter makes my blood boil. If it does the same to you, I would suggest turning the sound down in between programmes.

The brain is not designed to pass rapidly from a state of arousal to sleep, so anything exciting, annoying or upsetting is likely to delay the onset of sleep. The same is true of books; I would advise against thrillers at bedtime for this reason. Go for something less exciting: a magazine perhaps. For the past few years I have been reading *À la recherche du temps perdu* by Marcel Proust (in English – I'm terrible at languages) at the rate of half a page a night. It is a lovely book, beautifully written, with touches of soft humour, but nothing whatever happens in it and at around 6,000 pages I think that it should last longer than me.

A warning here – don't bring work home with you. You need at least a couple of hours relaxing or doing something useless before your brain will be ready to sleep.

Sex

This is sometimes a major source of discord between couples. After sex, most women become more alert while most men tend to fall asleep. This is due to the different effects of sexual intercourse on the nervous system of the two sexes and has become the source of many a gag for comedians, professional and amateur. For insomniac men (and occasionally women) this fact can be a useful point to take into account when considering the evening's agenda. Approach this carefully, though; an invitation such as 'How about it, then, because I want a good sleep' just won't do.

The repository of thoughts

You've had a very busy day; no time to think. I know it well. You get home late, have supper, have a chat and go to bed. At last you have the time and space to review the day and think what is needed for tomorrow. Suddenly you remember some essential task and you are worried that you will forget it by the morning. You work the problem through in your mind and it worries you because this problem throws up a whole load of others. How can you expect to sleep when you have programmed your brain to solve problems? The trouble is that if you try to exclude these thoughts from your mind they keep popping back. However hard you try, you can't clear your mind ready for slumber.

The brain is like that. It won't let something rest until it is sorted out or at least pigeon-holed. So pigeon-hole it. Keep a notepad by your bed. Every time a thought or problem comes into your head, write it down. Also write down a time in the morning when you will work out your plan to sort out each problem. For example:

7.30–8 a.m. sort out problems:

1 agenda for meeting;
2 sort out holiday arrangements;
3 phone bank manager about overdraft.

By putting your thoughts on paper, you take them out of your brain; but it will continue to worry unless you reassure it with a guarantee of a time when all will be made right. So when 7.30 a.m. comes, you must address your problem list, though it may well seem less important in the cold light of day.

Forgiveness

As I have said, many people use bedtime as a time to reflect on the day. You tend to focus on the annoying parts. You remember the incidents when someone was rude or somehow got one over on you. 'If only I had been quicker,' you muse, 'I could have made a stinging reply. That would have really put him in his place.' So you plan what devastating rejoinder you are going to throw at him tomorrow. All of this gets you quite worked up and, of course, you can't sleep.

The process is a complete waste of time, because never in the history of human experience has anyone been known to carry through the plan the next day. When the morning comes, it all seems trivial, and to seek the person out just to vent your spleen would be very silly. The fact is that in the darkness and solitude of the night, issues and feelings become magnified and only the next day do they resume realistic proportions.

So in order to sleep well the rule is that everyone is forgiven everything at night-time. This takes some practice but can be done. The next day, you can lay plans for murder if you wish; that is entirely your affair. But no recriminations at night.

Using these tips should improve your sleep. But if you are still ill with clinical depression, they won't work until you are quite a bit better. Just hold on; your sleep, like everything else, will improve with time.

Family and friends

It is a disappointing fact that it is usually those closest to you who treat you the worst when you are down. The reason is that they have come to rely on you. Your strength and reliability have long since become a given. Nobody thanks you for slaving away for them, as you have always done. People tend to organize their perceptions to suit themselves and to rationalize away their guilt. There is often no one more vindictive than someone in your debt, or more punishing than someone who is guilty.

To those of you recently recovered from clinical depression, I say this: don't waste time blaming your spouse or friends for neglecting your needs or for their lack of gratitude for all that you've done. Take responsibility for your own life, health and happiness. Nobody forced you to do what you do. Those around you put upon you *because you let them*. Now make another choice and take time and space for yourself. Don't expect them to be happy about it; they'll take time to adjust, but adjust they will. And what's more, you'll find they give you more too. The guilt and loss of self-esteem that results from giving up the role of 'she who will always provide' is temporary. The better balance in your life and the rewards this brings will be permanent.

Some partners remain supportive throughout the illness and the recovery process. These are great people, as it is pretty awful living through an episode of clinical depression in your nearest and dearest. Don't forget to acknowledge this when you get well. It has been a nightmare for you both, though it has been the fault of neither of you.

Conclusion:
What's the point?

I believe that one of the main secrets to getting the most out of life is to know what angers you. Express it, do what you can about it, then avoid the people and institutions that are responsible for generating it as much as you can. If you don't like where you are, then make another choice.

Most people are really quite good, most of the time. If that isn't your experience, you are letting the users of the world take too much of your life. They'll do that for as long as you let them, because they have a keen sense of who they can use and how much. The givers and doers, like you, will tend to collect these types. I would suggest you try to identify them and get them out of your life. Or if you are married to one, decide on your limits and boundaries, and stick to them.

The same applies to work. Most employers aren't abusive, but maybe you work for one that is. They select your type, and as other, less diligent employees leave quite quickly, you'll tend to find yourself increasingly alone in your plight. Unless, that is, you decide to take charge, stop being abused and change the way you operate, or if that is impossible, leave. You assume that no other employer will have you, but in fact you are an employer's dream. If you don't make a move, nothing will change; if you do, you are opting for a bit of risk and a lot of opportunity.

You see, life can certainly be better. Not that you can, or should, suddenly divest yourself of all your responsibilities. But if you decide that you are going to be responsible for yourself and your happiness, rather than being responsible for other people and theirs and then resenting the fact that nobody does the same for you, you'll be surprised how things can change. And then if you stop demanding that everyone approves of you all the time, or that life gives you what you seek instantly – now, that's exciting. Yes, this is true, even if you have three small children to look after, or are president of the World Bank.

You may feel that this way of thinking is selfish, or unchristian. I don't think it is. Is it better to give away your last seedlings to your hungry brothers to eat now, or to plant them, so that they, you and many others may thrive in the future? I suggest that even you don't know how much good you'll be able to do if you stay well.

You and I have made plenty of mistakes, but please don't condemn yourself for not having had hindsight when you made yours. The episode from which you, or someone close to you, have, hopefully, emerged was an opportunity, terrible though it was. You have confronted the fact that, in your headlong pursuit of excellence or your life's work of trying to please everyone, you missed the point. In fact, though, you have learnt what you never could have done had you or those around you remained well. Come on – you know it's true. You wouldn't have stopped and re-evaluated your life had you not been stopped dead in your tracks. A certain Roman citizen on the road to Damascus comes to mind. Now that it has happened, just make sure you change; if you do, I've got good news for you: you've found the key to a happier life.

The world has goodness, kindness and fun mixed in with the badness, cruelty and oppression. Your task is to sort out the one from the other, while accepting your body's design limits. If you don't overload the fuse, it won't blow; if you do, it will. It's your choice.

In any case, you can't achieve that much, whatever you do. Mother Teresa of Calcutta got it right: 'We cannot achieve great things on this earth, we can only do small things with great love.' Pace yourself while you do them. Find time to stop and smell the flowers. Or in the words of two of my wisest patients, 'However busy, stressed and late you are, don't walk up escalators.'